P9-CEH-828

Fantastic Flax

A powerful defense against cancer, heart disease and digestive disorders

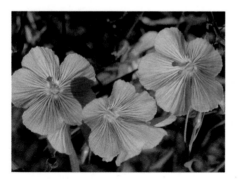

Siegfried Gursche

alive
books

Vancouver
Canada

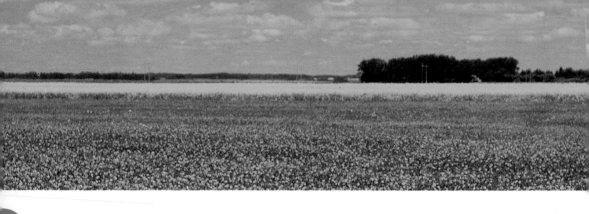

Contents

All About Flax

Delicious Flax Recipes

IMPORTANT

It is your constitutional right to educate yourself in health and medical knowledge, to seek helpful information and make use of it for your own benefit, and for that of your family. You are the one responsible for your health. In order to make decisions in all health matters, you must educate yourself. Share the contents of this book with your certified health practitioner and make sure you inform him or her that you are changing your diet and lifestyle.

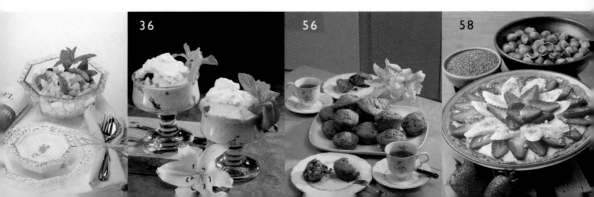

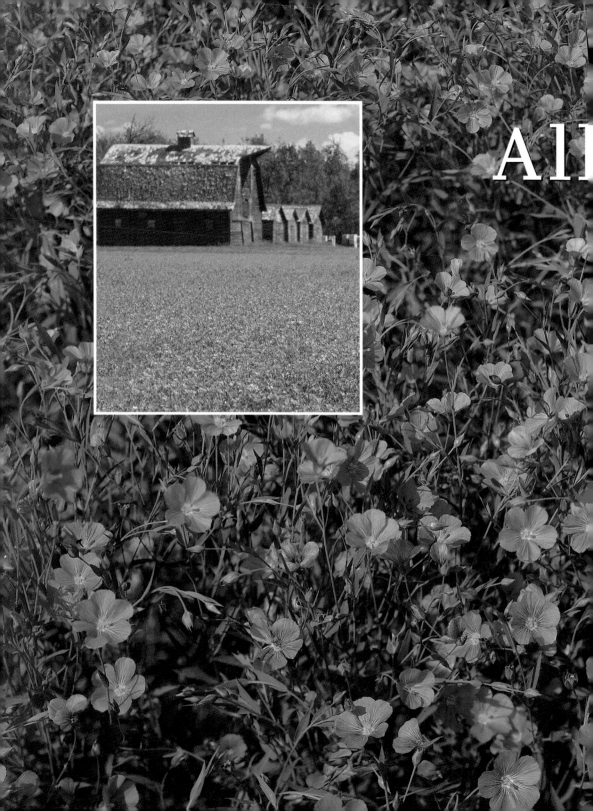

Al

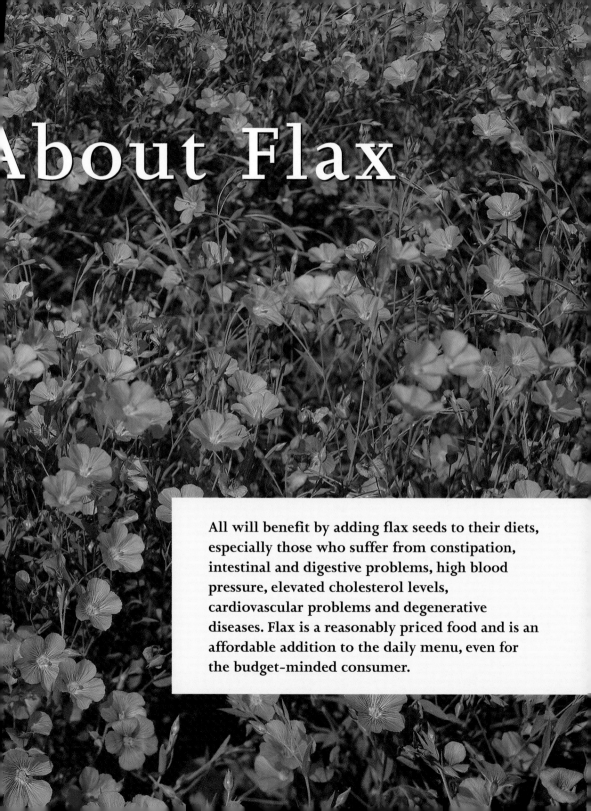

About Flax

All will benefit by adding flax seeds to their diets, especially those who suffer from constipation, intestinal and digestive problems, high blood pressure, elevated cholesterol levels, cardiovascular problems and degenerative diseases. Flax is a reasonably priced food and is an affordable addition to the daily menu, even for the budget-minded consumer.

Introduction

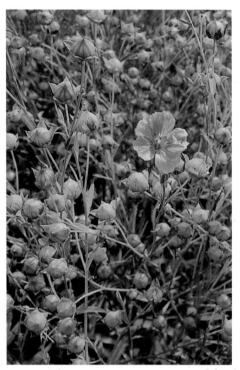

These flax husks are getting ready for harvest.

Flax is a nutritional powerhouse and a super healing food. It is an ancient but little-known seed whose benefits have only recently been recognized in North America by nutritionists, dietitians and naturopathic doctors. Even in orthodox medical circles it has gained attention and is now being studied as a "nutraceutical" – a food with many nutrients and pharmaceutical properties. The empirical evidence, which for thousands of years has shown flax to be a healing food, has recently been substantiated in clinical studies at universities and hospitals around the world. For example, the University of Toronto recently published studies conducted by Dr. Stephen Cunnane, who showed that flax prevents the growth of new cancer cells and lowers blood cholesterol levels. At a recent convention on experimental biology, the American Food and Drug Agency endorsed flax seeds as a food for disease prevention. Without a doubt, flax has a promising future and a great place in human nutrition as a healing food and nutraceutical. Everyone will benefit by adding flax seeds to their diet, especially those who suffer from constipation, intestinal and digestive problems, high blood pressure, elevated cholesterol levels, cardiovascular problems and degenerative diseases. Flax is reasonably priced and is an affordable addition to the daily diet, even for the budget-minded consumer.

My first encounter with flax, or linseed as we called it, was when I was eleven. I spent a summer and fall with my grandfather on his small farm in eastern Germany. He had about thirty-six acres of land, with four cows, two horses, a flock of geese, ducks and chickens. It was 1944, the year before World War II ended. Food was generally scarce and farmers tried to be self-sufficient by growing a wide variety of foods including potatoes, vegetables, all kinds of grains (barley, rye and wheat for baking their own bread, and oats for the horses) and flax. I still remember the field of blue flax in bloom the day I arrived at the farm. It was an unforgettable sight.

Farmers grew flax for several reasons. The fiber of the plant stems was processed and spun into a yarn used for weaving fine linen; hence the name "linseed." My grandmother loved to work with flax fiber. The strands of fiber were very long and she spun them on her simple spinning wheel into a thin and even thread that was much finer than wool. To this day fine linen tablecloths, sheets and clothes are treasured for their beauty, texture and durability.

Farmers know how to use flax seeds to treat many diseases and keep their animals healthy. So do veterinarians. My father, who grew up on this small farm, was responsible for brushing the horses. He observed that flax-fed horses had much shinier coats than those that didn't and this made his job easier.

Flax is a boon to farmers for other reasons as well. The small, hard seeds soak up eight times their weight in water. Nature has made it that way so that the kernel, when seeded, can store enough moisture to sprout and grow, even if after the first rain there is a lengthy dry spell. In the United States, Canada, Australia and Eastern Europe, where most of the world's flax is grown today, farmers often face dry spells after the seed has been put into the ground without worrying that their flax won't grow.

I remember one day my grandfather rushed into the storage room with a bucket of hot water, grabbed a few handfuls of flax seeds and mixed them into the water. "There is trouble with the cow," he said. "I let her out of the barn too early after the rain and she ate too much wet grass." (Cows who eat large amounts of wet grass will experience bloating.) "This flax will fix her in no time! All that's needed is that the seeds soak up the water in the next half hour." And, sure enough, within half an hour the flax and water turned into a warm slurry mash which the cow slurped up happily.

This ability of the kernels to soak up an incredible amount

The flax plant has a variety of uses. It provides food and medicine for humans and animals, and the flax fibers can be spun into linen for clothing.

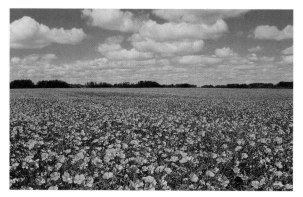

of water and turn it into mucilage (a glutinous liquid) has also provided people with gentle relief from all kinds of gastrointestinal discomfort, congestion and constipation for thousands of years. Flax mucilage is an excellent remedy for stomach ulcers, as it covers the inflamed areas and protects them from the stomach acids. Because flax is very alkaline, it also helps to prevent heartburn and should be included in all detoxification programs to restore the body's proper acid-alkaline balance.

There are many more wonderful things to be said about flax. Some you may already know, others may be new for you. While the facts about flax are no longer secret, the many health benefits are still widely unknown.

Flax Seed – Food or Drug? . . . .

Flax is an oil-bearing seed. It contains the highest percentage of both "essential fats" – which are linolenic acid (an omega-3 fatty acid) and linoleic acid (an omega-6 fatty acid) – of any oil-bearing seed. The essential fats are necessary for the proper function of many organs, however they are not produced by the body. The essential fats, therefore, must be supplied by the diet. These are the "healing fats" Udo Erasmus talks about in detail in his book *Fats that Heal, Fats that Kill*. The essential fats are good for you and will not make you fat, so you don't have to worry about calories when you eat foods that contain a lot of essential fats. The main purpose of these two essential fatty acids is not to provide energy or to store fat in the body. Instead, they supply the body with hormone-like substances called prostaglandins and eicosanoids, which ensure the proper function of the brain, nervous system, skin and sexual organs. They also prevent blood platelets from becoming sticky and forming blood clots; in other words, they keep the blood thin thereby controlling high blood pressure. The scientist H.M. Sinclair

"Flax oil is the spark plug that cranks up fat metabolism in our bodies."
– Johanna Budwig

8

reported in 1984 that after putting himself on an experimental diet high in omega-3, he noticed striking changes taking place in his body. First he lost weight, then his energy level increased and he experienced more vitality than ever! Dr. Johanna Budwig, a pioneer in the field of health and nutrition research, explains: "Flax oil is the spark plug that cranks up fat metabolism in our bodies." The health benefits of flax seeds are overwhelming and we will take a closer look at them a little later in this book.

Flax Has a Long History . . . .

Flax seeds have been part of the human diet for over five thousand years. Records tell us that in ancient Babylon (3000 BC) flax was already cultivated for food. One thousand years later a complex irrigation system along the Euphrates and Tigris rivers was developed, mainly to ensure a rich harvest of flax.

The famed Greek physician Hippocrates (460–377 BC), known as the father of natural medicine, recognized flax as a food which relieves intestinal discomfort. He coined the often quoted, now proverbial phrase, "Let food be your medicine and your medicine be your food." There is probably no better commodity than flax that fits both categories "food" and "medicine."

Charlemagne (AD 742–814), King of the Franks and Holy Roman Emperor, established laws in his medical law book *Capitulare*, governing the cultivation of flax for food and medicinal purposes. Because of the unique properties of flax seeds, their high nutrient and fiber content, he considered them tremendously important as cleansers and relievers of gastrointestinal problems.

© Roberto Hernandez

Hippocrates considered illness to be a natural phenomenon that forced people to discover the imbalances in their health.

Flax has been widely used in Europe as a staple food for centuries. The seeds store well and provide good nourishment in lean times. Today, you will have a hard time finding any bakery in Germany that does not bake a flax-rye bread. The oil from the flax seeds adds moisture to the bread, thereby extending its shelf-life and improving its texture. Whenever I travel to Germany I'm astonished to see the variety of breads and buns baked with flax. The Flax Council of Canada reports that in

Germany over 60,000 tons of flax seed are consumed annually in bread and cereal. On average, that amounts to about two and a half pounds (one kilogram) per person per year or one teaspoon (three grams) daily. Current consumption levels of flax seed by Canadians are low enough that Statistics Canada does not yet document them as it does many other, more common foods. However, the stage is set for a change.

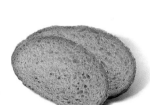

Mucilage . . . .

Why does flax work so well as a laxative? It all has to do with the hard shell which makes up twelve per cent of the seed. As soon as this shell comes in contact with moisture it absorbs it quickly and expands into a glutinous liquid known as mucilage. Two tablespoons (thirty grams) of flax seed stirred into a glass of boiling hot water will thicken up quickly and have the consistency of a pudding. To use flax as a laxative, drink the mix before it thickens up; the thickening will then happen in the stomach. If constipation persists, drink a glass of water with two tablespoons (thirty grams) of whole flax seeds twice daily before meals. By the way, the unbroken flax seed, protected by the shell, will pass right through the digestive system without breaking down. Our bodies can only digest flax seeds and benefit from their many nutritional qualities if the shell is broken.

Our bodies can only digest flax seeds and benefit from their many nutritional qualities if the shell is broken.

The flax mucilage can also serve another important purpose; namely, to repair the damage caused by taking massive doses of antibiotics. The friendly bacteria in your intestines are destroyed in large quantities if you take antibiotics, birth control pills or other drugs such as those used in chemotherapy, particularly over a long period of time, and chronic constipation (common among hospital patients) may develop. Flax mucilage helps the intestinal flora to re-establish itself. Dr. Ernst Schneider, author of many books on natural health, agrees: "From my previous experience, the intestinal flora recovers more quickly from a chemotherapeutic shock if freshly crushed flax is consumed regularly." The mucilage from flax helps to repair any damage to the internal "wallpaper," which is the coating of mucus that lines the entire digestive tract. Even people who suffer from stomach ulcers will heal better and faster by eating flax because the mucilage covers the inflamed areas and protects them from the stomach acid.

Fiber . . . .

Sixty years ago, scientists began to study the effects of food fiber on human health. At first, scientists believed that fiber had no nutritional value and was therefore unimportant in any food or diet. That is why, in the milling process, bran (which is all fiber) was removed from the grain, leaving behind only white, starchy flour stripped of all vitamins and minerals. Then researchers began looking at the diets of people who lived in underdeveloped countries. These people typically ate high-fiber diets and did not experience constipation and other kinds of disorders, like Crohn's disease, diverticulitis and high cholesterol, that are rampant in all industrialized nations. All of a sudden, fiber was a medical buzzword. In flax seeds, fiber is the structural material of the shells and the substance in which the oil is embedded. Humans cannot digest it but the friendly bacteria or micro-organisms thriving in the intestines can and they use it for energy.

Consuming flax seed regularly will lower cholesterol level and blood pressure.

Like many other foods, flax has two types of fiber: soluble and insoluble. Two-thirds of the fiber in flax is insoluble, consisting of cellulose and lignin. This fiber cleans out the intestines like a broom, reducing the bowel transit time by passing fecal matter rapidly. The other one-third of fiber is water soluble and plays an important role in

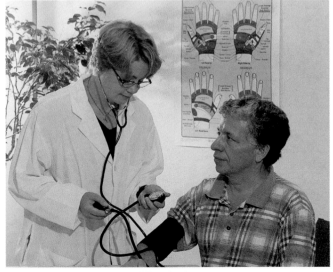

reducing serum cholesterol levels and regulating blood glucose levels. This is good news for people with diabetes. The British

Journal of Nutrition confirmed these positive effects on persons consuming flax seeds daily during a four-week study. The blood glucose levels of the people in the study group were reduced by twenty-seven per cent, while their cholesterol levels were reduced by seven per cent. In all cases their bowel movements improved. This is important because fecal matter that lingers in the intestines creates harmful compounds and toxins. This can cause serious illness and even cancer of the colon. In fact, the National Cancer Institute has officially recognized fiber as an important element in the diet for the prevention of many cancers.

Lignans . . . .

Not only do lignans prevent some cancers but they also play an important role in maintaining healthy, strong bones.

Not too long ago the word "lignan" could not be found in any medical dictionary. Lignans are an important, newly discovered group of substances. They are plant estrogens (phytoestrogens) that may play a key role in the prevention of breast, prostate, uterus and colon cancers. These friendly plant hormones not only prevent some cancers but they also play an important role in maintaining healthy, strong bones. Lignans also prevent the formation of gallstones by binding with bile acids. According to the research of Dr. L. Thompson of the University of Toronto, flax seeds are the richest source of lignans and contain 75 to 800 times more than wheat bran, oats, millet, rye, legumes, soybeans and 66 other plant foods tested.

Lignans also protect the body from estrogen-driven cancers by expelling excess estrogen from the body and by interfering with tumor cell growth. It is well established that Mexican, Japanese and Chinese women, whose diets are high in fiber and lignans, are far less likely to develop breast cancer than women eating the standard North American diet. What is more, lignans attach themselves to estrogen receptor sites and take the place of estradiol and estrone, which are implicated in breast cancer. Lignans also inhibit estrogen production from fatty tissue. Many studies support the contention that people who consume high amounts of flax with lignans are able to balance the hormone levels in their body.

Furthermore, researchers believe that lignans may help treat or prevent the following conditions: heart disease, diabetes, high blood pressure and possibly asthma. Finally, lignans have anti-bacterial, anti-viral and anti-fungal properties and this makes flax a powerful immune system booster.

The Wonder Grain . . . .

Flax seed has some additional healthy ingredients, which makes it an excellent whole food for humans. It contains vitamins A, B_1, B_2, C, D and E; a full array of minerals and trace minerals, carotene, lecithin and phospholipids. The oil content of the seed is thirty-five to forty-five per cent and of course it has plenty of fiber and protein. It should be noted that the composition varies from one variety of seed to another and is dependent on climatic conditions. For example, one growing season may have ideal weather conditions yielding a perfect crop, while a rainy and cold summer may produce meagre seeds. Flax is the ideal survival food. Everything is well protected within a hard shell with antioxidants (such as vitamins C and E, and beta carotene) that will keep the seed fresh for many years. Only when the shell is broken and the oil is exposed to oxygen will the oil spoil and turn rancid.

An Almost Perfect Protein . . . .

It is a little-known fact that flax provides a high quality, though not complete protein. (It is not complete because there are several amino acids which are present only in insignificant amounts.) The amino acids that make up the protein in flax combine extremely well with those contained in milk or any of its products such as yogurt, kefir, buttermilk or cottage cheese. Together, these amino acids form a complete protein, which the body finds much easier to digest than a partial protein. This is good news not only for vegetarians, but for everybody!

The following chart shows the findings of Dr. J. Schormüller of the University of Technology in Berlin. It compares the amount of different amino acids in several foods, including whole egg protein, the food that contains the highest

Amino Acid Profile of Flax, Milk and Eggs				
Essential Amino Acids	**Flax Protein**	**Milk Protein**	**Whole Egg Protein**	**Desirable Daily Intake**
Isoleucine	4.0%	6.2%	10.2%	1.4%
Leucine	7.0	11.3	18.3	2.2
Lysine	3.8	7.5	11.3	1.6
Methionine	2.3	3.3	5.6	2.2
Phenylalanine	5.6	5.3	10.9	2.2
Threonine	5.1	4.6	9.7	1.0
Tryptophan	1.9	1.6	3.5	1.0
Valine	7.0	6.6	13.6	1.6

amount of usable protein. There are fifteen amino acids. The ones shown here are only the *essential* ones.

In his report *Linseeds as Food*, Dr. Schormüller states: "Forty grams (one and a half ounces) of a mixture consisting of equal parts of linseeds and milk will provide all the essential amino acids in sufficient amounts and in a desirable ratio to one another." In comparison to any other source of protein, such as milk, cheese, fish, eggs or meat, you will find flax seeds to be an inexpensive yet valuable source of quality protein. Canadian-grown brown flax contains twenty-four per cent protein, while golden flax contains twenty-eight per cent.

Interesting Discoveries . . . .

In the late 70s and early 80s, I was involved in extensive research for the development of marketable flax products, including a stable cracked flax seed and, of course, cold-pressed, unrefined fresh flax oil. I traveled the Canadian prairies, meeting flax growers. In Vulcan, south of Calgary, I met

Russel Smith, a farmer cultivating many acres of organic flax. We looked at all popular varieties of brown flax – about six different kinds. It was here that I saw for the first time three different kinds of golden (or yellow) flax. The kernels of the golden flax were generally larger, slightly softer and, in my opinion, tastier than the brown ones.

Russel explained that golden flax is usually a little more expensive than brown flax. The reason is that the harvest yield per acre is much less than brown flax. Golden flax has a higher protein content but it does not yield as much oil. That is why yellow flax is not used for pressing oils but is used for cereals and baking bread. He informed me that plant breeders in Morden, Manitoba were involved in a cooperative agreement with Agriculture Canada, and were developing a strain of yellow flax that yielded a lot of oil but very little omega-3. Australian plant breeders had already developed a genetically modified variety of yellow flax with dramatically reduced levels of omega-3. The aim of this project was to create a strain of flax which

Cost comparison of protein from different food sources		
Food	Cost per 32 oz (1000 g)	Per cent of protein	Cost of protein per 3.2 oz (100 g)
Lean ground meat	$34.20	19.3%	$17.78
Chicken, meat only	14.31	21.4	6.68
Farmed salmon	21.50	21.3	10.09
Whole fresh eggs	2.08	12.5	1.67
Milk, 3.25% butter fat	1.29	3.3	3.90
Cottage cheese	9.98	12.5	7.95
Gouda cheese	17.90	22.7	7.88
Gruyère cheese	24.90	25.6	9.72
Cheddar cheese	13.90	25.0	5.56
Flax - Canadian, yellow	2.90	25.0	1.19
Flax - US, brown	2.45	19.3	1.27

Note: Prices are given in Canadian currency.

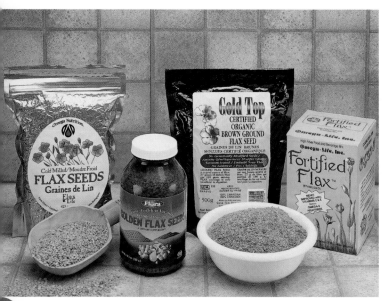

Flax meal sold in vacuum-sealed foil packages is a convenient way to use flax. Once open, refrigerate and use within two weeks.

would not turn rancid thereby extending its shelf-life and making it suitable as a cooking oil.

In May 1993, Health and Welfare Canada gave its approval to market the "refined" linola™ oil in Canada which is an oil produced from this genetically engineered seed. Here is another example of industry, motivated by financial gain, tinkering with nature in order to produce an oil where the most healthy ingredient (omega-3) is eliminated. While the shelf-life of this product is extended, it will not extend the span of a human life.

The original golden seeds we worked with are very nutritious and today are used mostly as cereal. To be used for a cereal the seeds needed to be processed in such a way that the stomach juices could penetrate the seeds and digest them without opening oil cells. They needed to be intact to avoid oxygenation and rancidity. In our experiments, golden flax was most suitable when crushed slightly, not cracked or milled – just squeezed enough to break the shell open without damaging the oil cells. In this way the kernels can be used as ready-made cereal, and are able to absorb liquids from yogurt, kefir or milk. They could also be sprinkled on porridge without the oil turning rancid. We coined this edible golden flax product "Linoseed", which I personally prefer to brown flax for breakfast muesli. Milled flax or flax meal from brown flax, loosely packaged in plastic bags, used to be very popular in the 1970s and is still sold in some health food stores today. Dr. Paavo Airola, the nation's leading nutritionist at that time, warned consumers not to purchase flax meal or ground flax, as the exposed oil in ground flax oxidizes rapidly and goes rancid within days. Heat, light and air all contribute to this process of oxidization. Rancid oils should be avoided as they are toxic and cancer-causing. Today, however, some companies offer specially milled flax seeds in vacuum-sealed foil packages. They utilize a unique new milling technique and can guarantee freshness. If you would like to try these products, make sure that the production date is no more than three months before the purchase date and once the package is opened, refrigerate it, keep the bag tightly closed and consume it within two weeks.

Another interesting discovery we made was that varieties of flax grown in colder regions, such as Saskatchewan or the Peace River region in northern Alberta, contain proportionally more omega-3 linolenic fatty acids and less omega-6 linoleic fatty acids than varieties grown in warmer climates, such as the midwest of the United States. This phenomenon was also reflected in the taste, as colder climate flax produced a slightly bitter and stronger flavor.

Flax seed is probably the most economical source of any protein (see chart on page 15).

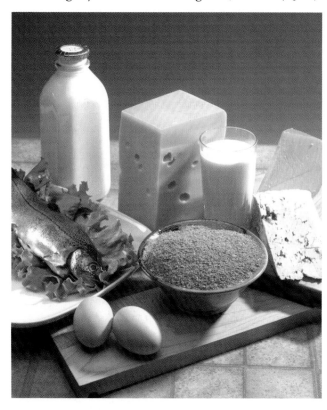

It is interesting to note that nature takes care of the people up north who obviously need more omega-3 in their oils, which stay liquid even in freezing temperatures. Oil seeds, like sunflower or safflower grown in warmer regions have only traces of omega-3, while sesame, almond or olive oil, as well as all tropical oils, such as coconut, palm, avocado, macadamia and Brazil nut oils, have no omega-3 at all. Yet people living in the tropics consuming tropical oils without omega-3 and little omega-6 still do well without showing any symptoms of fat-related

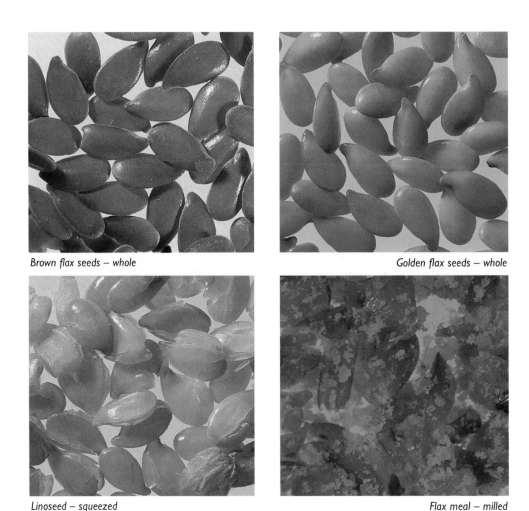

Brown flax seeds – whole

Golden flax seeds – whole

Linoseed – squeezed

Flax meal – milled

degenerative diseases. The secret is obviously that populations living in the tropics consume their coconut and palm oils in unrefined, natural states. Once these people adopt a diet including refined, heat-damaged vegetable oils, they show the same symptoms of degenerative diseases that are rampant in industrialized nations.

Flax has so much to offer! It is unequaled in versatility as a therapeutic plant and as a nourishing food. As a matter of fact, flax seeds could be called "the Golden Miracle Workers." Consider them when you are thinking about your health and that of your family.

Flax Oil . . . .

It just wouldn't be right to talk about all the health benefits of flax seeds and not mention the oils pressed from flax seeds. Flax oil is in a class of its own, simply because it is the only oil that is made up almost entirely of very good poly-unsaturated essential fatty acids. Essential means that the fatty acids are required by the body to stay healthy; they need to come from food sources because the body cannot produce them on its own. Poly-unsaturated oils are "hungry" for oxygen and this is the reason why they go rancid so quickly. They also dry fast, which is why linseed oil is used for paint.

Flax seed contains forty-two per cent oil. When expeller pressed in a cold process, the yield is about thirty-three per cent oil. This oil is made up of forty-eight to sixty-four per cent of linolenic fatty acids (omega-3-LNA) which makes flax the richest source by far. Sixteen to thirty-four per cent of the oil is comprised of linoleic fatty acids (omega-6-LA) and the balance (eighteen per cent) is mostly oleic fatty acids (omega-9), a mono-unsaturated but not essential fatty acid that is found in large quantities in olive oil.

Since flax oil is poly-unsaturated, with the main component being omega-3, it spoils fast when heated or exposed to oxygen and light. You want to use it for cold dishes, in salad dressings for all kinds of green salads, potato salad, grated carrot salad, coleslaw or with raw sauerkraut. Freshly pressed, unrefined flax oil is delicious when poured over a baked potato with some herbal salt. I love it.

The great comeback of flax oil was initiated by Dr. Johanna Budwig with her famous oil-protein diet for cancer patients and others suffering from cardiovascular

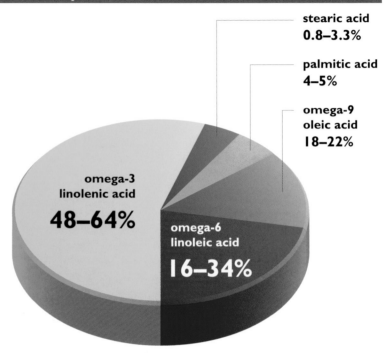

stearic acid 0.8–3.3%

palmitic acid 4–5%

omega-9 oleic acid 18–22%

Flax oil is the highest single source for omega-3 fatty acid

omega-3 linolenic acid

48–64%

omega-6 linoleic acid

16–34%

disease, arthritis and other degenerative diseases. The recipe consisted mainly of flax oil mixed into quark (a soft spreadable cheese made by straining warmed-up kefir, yogurt or buttermilk), a grated apple and freshly ground flax seeds (see recipe section for *Budwig Muesli*).

I visited Dr. Johanna Budwig on two occasions while traveling in Germany. She was a fascinating person to talk with. Dr. Budwig was a pioneering scientist in the field of health and nutrition.

Her greatest contribution was the isolation and identification of fatty substances in the blood. She was the first scientist to analyze the different fatty acids through gas and paper chromophotography, making it possible to determine good fats from bad fats. Dr. Budwig denounced the margarine manufacturers' methods of turning good unrefined healthy oils into highly processed and hydrogenated health-endangering margarine.

Dr. Budwig concluded that fresh unrefined flax oil had the

best health-giving profile provided it was not heated. Heating flax oil and other poly-unsaturated fats turn the good "cis-form" of the fatty acids into the bad "trans-form."

Dr. Budwig recounted her achievements and also her many struggles. The orthodox medical establishment, the margarine manufacturers and the government all opposed her in one way or another and attempted to suppress her findings by prosecuting her for claiming that trans-fatty acids and the hydrogenation process are harmful to humans. Dr. Budwig maintained that the process of artificially hardening liquid vegetable oils (hydrogenation) creates life-threatening fat molecules – the trans-fatty acids. The industry disagreed and took her to court. She fought twenty-eight court cases in her life and won all of them. Today, it is widely accepted that trans-fatty acids are the cause of certain cancers, heart disease and a host of other degenerative diseases.

When choosing flax oil, or any edible oil for that matter, be very, very careful. Not all manufacturers offer a high-quality product and deliver what the label promises. Before I was involved in setting up an oil pressing plant in Vancouver, my wife and I traveled to Europe and visited a number of oil mills, where so-called cold-pressed oils were produced. We visited East Germany's most productive flax oil mill in Halberstadt; we saw the old oil mill in Künzelsau and looked at a great number of modern oil presses. What we saw was not nice. Nor were we impressed with the large-volume oil presses in Saskatoon or San Francisco. They all used outdated huge platen or expeller presses which produced considerable heat in the pressing process. The oil they produced was unpalatable and in need of further refining. Their labels, however, read "cold-pressed" or "expeller-pressed," always hiding the fact that the oil was refined. The government does not require manufacturers to declare on the label that an oil has been refined. Yet the refining process requires a high temperature which changes the molecular structure of flax oil from the cis- to the trans-form.

We wanted to produce truly cold-pressed, unrefined fresh-tasting flax oil and found the suitable presses in Germany. Of course, they were running slowly and could press only small amounts but they made delicious oil. With the proper packaging and bottling equipment (which would keep light and oxy-

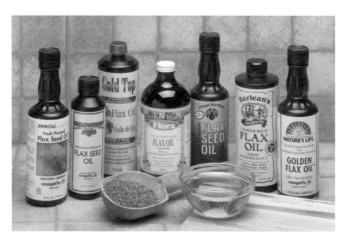

Always purchase unrefined oils. Make sure they are packaged in dark containers as light will damage oils. You will find these oils in the refrigerator department of health food stores.

gen out) our company was the first to supply North America with true, fresh cold-pressed and unrefined flax oil. Today, there are at least six reliable companies in Canada and the US that press the oil the way we did and the result is a variety of healthy healing oils for the consumer.

The label information you need to look for is a statement including the words "cold expeller-pressed" and most importantly, "unrefined." You should also see a pressing date; do not purchase flax oil after six months past the pressing date. Rather, buy small (8.5 oz or 250 ml bottles) and consume the oil within three weeks after opening rather than buying larger bottles just to save money. One more thing: beware of supermarket oils. Other than extra-virgin and virgin olive oils and those just mentioned, all oils are refined and heat-treated and contain the dangerous trans-fatty acids. The government does not require oil manufactures to declare the percentage of trans-fatty acids on the label. Once vegetable oils have undergone the heat-refining process, heat-damaged fat molecules, trans-fatty acids, are present.

How to Use Flax . . . .

All health food stores carry flax seeds, which are sometimes packaged on the premises in small, medium and large bags. It is most economical to purchase flax in bulk and store the seeds in canisters in a dry place at home. The most common are the smaller shiny reddish-brown colored seeds. They are flat and oval with pointed tips, slightly larger than sesame seeds and have a nutty flavor. Some stores also carry the golden or yellow variety or may bring them in for you upon request. These seeds are slightly larger and a little softer, making them perfect for cereal.

Benefits of Eating Flax Seeds and Oil

Biochemical Effect	Clinical Result
Normalizes the body's fatty acids	Smoother skin, shiny hair, soft hands; increased stamina, vitality and agility
Normalizes and rebalances prostaglandins	Smoother muscle action; improvement of many other functions; alleviates adverse symptoms of PMS and menopause
Reduces appetite provocation, lowers glycemic index of foods and slows down glucose absorption	Eliminates binging or addictive need for carbohydrate-rich foods
Stabilizes insulin and blood sugar levels	Prevents high-sugar-low-sugar blues; keeps stamina high for long periods
Strengthens the immune system	Avoids or overcomes food allergies; fights off some diseases more effectively
Increases fiber and aerobic bacteria	Promotes proper functioning of the bacteria in the digestive tract to avoid gas, constipation and other disorders leading to diverticulitis and Crown's disease
Normalizes blood fats and lowers cholesterol	Stronger cardiovascular system; clear thinking
Corrects the body's thermogenic system	Burns off fat (ability to burn off calories); cold-weather resistance; increases comfort
Elevates the level of estrogen in blood	Dramatically reduces many post-menopausal plasma in post-menopausal women symptoms
Supports liver in fat metabolism	Lowers or normalizes blood pressure

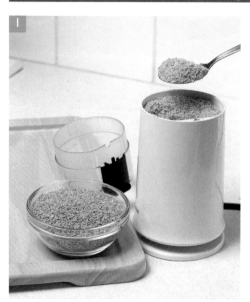

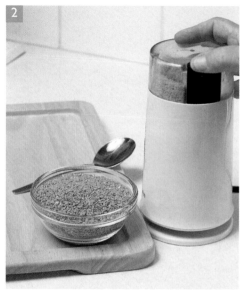

1 To grind your own flax seeds, put up to four tbsp seeds in an electric coffee grinder.

2 For cracked flax, grind for two seconds only.

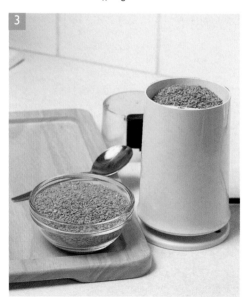

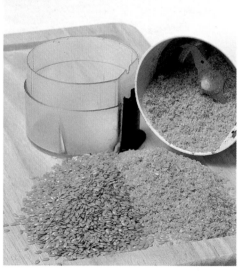

3 For fine flax meal grind for six seconds.

4 Vary the texture of your meals by adding either cracked flax seeds or fine flax meal.

The best way to integrate flax into your diet is in its raw form. The recommended portion is one tablespoon per day. For grinding the seeds I recommend obtaining an electric coffee grinder like those made by Braun, Salton or Philips. They can be bought anywhere for under $20 and do a wonderful job grinding the seeds. Do not attempt to grind flax in a regular flour mill. The seeds, with their high oil content, will quickly plug up the grinding stones. A blender could work also, but it's rather big for such a small job. Using an electric coffee grinder, pulse the seeds for just two seconds – not longer. This will turn the seeds into a coarse powder, ready to use.

Breakfast You can stir the flax powder into porridge, cooked multi-grain cereal or, the way I like it best, mixed into a bowl of kefir, buttermilk or plain natural yogurt. There are many other ways to use freshly ground raw flax which you will find in the recipe section. Eating flax seeds raw will provide you with their total food value including the protein, essential fats and the lignans.

Soups You can even derive benefits from cooked flax seeds. All you have to do is to add one or two tablespoons of seeds to two or three cups of water and bring the mixture to a boil. Remove from the heat, strain the mucilage then mix it into soups, sauces, vegetable or grain dishes. Naturally, a few spoonfuls of ground seeds can be added to vegetable broth to thicken it or make a soup more creamy. Remember not to boil ground flax, just add the ground flax after the boiling soup has been removed from the heat and let stand for five minutes before serving. For soups I actually like the ground golden flax – it looks better. I have a vegan friend who soaks flax seeds in water, stirs them through a strainer and uses the gel in recipes whenever eggs are called for.

Dessert The most exciting cooked flax recipe I know is called *Rumpelstiltskin*. In the recipe section you will find the instructions for making this most delicious pudding. My wife Christel has presented the dish at many different health-oriented functions, including the Emerald Lake Health Retreats and several health food conventions. She has even shared the recipe with the chefs of famous hotels such as the Royal York in Toronto, the Hyatt Regency in Vancouver, the Harrison Hot Springs Resort and the

Hotel Vancouver. Sometimes she received doubting looks, but once the concoction was finished the chefs approved and were excited. One of the European chefs commented, "This is exactly what my grandmother used to serve us kids, and we loved it." *Rumpelstiltskin* was always a crowning success and a satisfying way to finish an excellent meal. At social functions it became a tradition to serve it. I remember one banquet where *Rumpelstiltskin* was not served at dessert. The guests revolted and while pounding their hands on the table they chanted: "We want Rumpelstiltskin, we want Rumpelstiltskin!" Whenever Christel served this incredible dessert at sales meetings or other company gatherings there were always requests for seconds. You must try it!

Bread baking As mentioned earlier, flax can be used in breads, buns and muffins. Some recipes in the recipe section call for whole flax seeds in the European tradition and others for flax meal or a mixture of both. Whole seeds should always be soaked in water for at least an hour before using them in a recipe that calls for baking. I have often been asked "What about the heat – doesn't it harm the omega-3 and -6?" This is certainly a valid question and the answer is – no, the essential fats will be unharmed. (There wouldn't be a problem inside the bread because of the moisture. However the seeds on the crust would be spoiled.) As you may remember from your high school chemistry class, the temperature of water does not rise beyond 212°F (100°C), unless under pressure. In other words, the water absorbed by the seeds keeps the oil from overheating. When you bake bread you can replace ten to thirty per cent of the flour with flax meal. As the proportion of ground flax seed increases, the baked volume decreases, resulting in a firmer loaf.

Baking will not harm the essential fatty acids in flax seeds provided they have been soaked beforehand.

Flax bread made with ripe bubbling kefir is heaven on earth. The kefir enhances the taste of flax bread immensely. The nutty flavor of flax seeds also enhances the taste of pancakes, muffins and waffles, which can also be made with kefir to make them taste even better.

Skincare Flax seeds can even be helpful in skin cleansing programs and are especially effective in normalizing oily, dry or blemished skin. Young people with problem skin will find this to be much more helpful than relying on harsh chemical compounds. This mask stimulates the circulation and leaves your skin feeling soft and smooth. To make the mildly abrasive skin cleanser, mix equal parts of freshly ground flax seeds and wheat bran, take two tablespoons of the mixture and stir in enough hot water to make a paste.

The flax facial mask

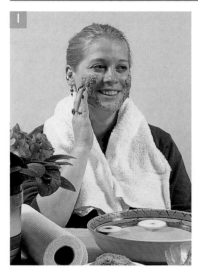

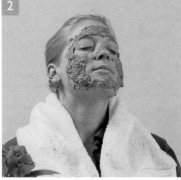

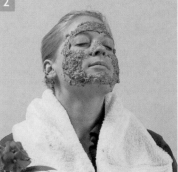

2 Leave the mask on for five to ten minutes. During this time the ground flax seeds will lubricate your skin and provide it with essential fatty acids, which can help to relieve dryness.

3 Rinse your face with water. This is a safe and gentle procedure that can be used every day in place of soap. It can even be used as a body scrub.

1 Moisten your face with water, then gently massage the mix on your skin with a circular motion.

Finally, cracked flax makes a very good poultice for sore and bruised muscles as well as inflamed tissues. The poultice also brings relief for rheumatic pains and neuralgia. Skin conditions such as wounds, boils, ulcerations and inflammations benefit from repeated flax poultice applications. Internal inflammations, such as bursitis, gastric inflammation, cystitis, and kidney stone and gallstone formation can be alleviated by regularly applying a poultice. It's easy to make, just follow these simple instructions.

Making a flax poultice

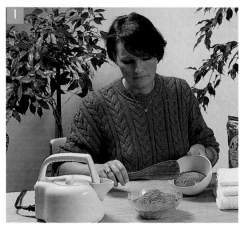

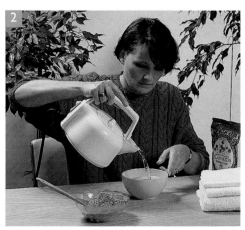

1 Measure one cup of ground flax seeds into a bowl.

2 Add one cup of hot water and let sit for ten minutes.

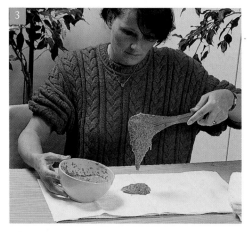

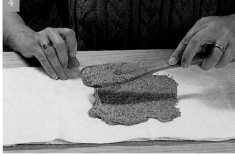

3 – 4 Spread the mixture evenly over the middle of a linen cloth.

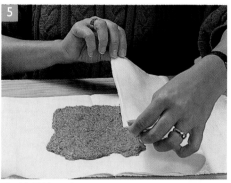

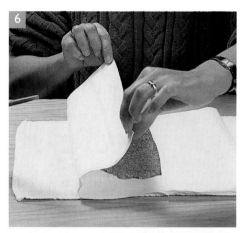

5 – 7 Fold as shown.

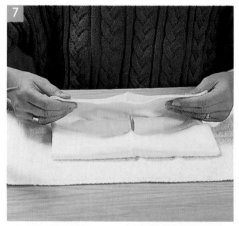

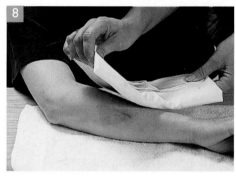

8 – 10 Apply to affected area and wrap with a clean dry towel. Leave the poultice on for two to three hours or overnight.

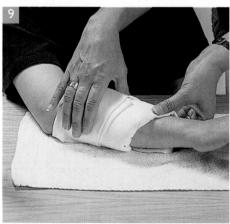

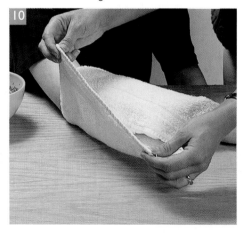

Delicious Flax

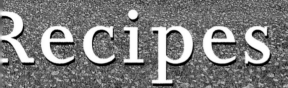

Recipes

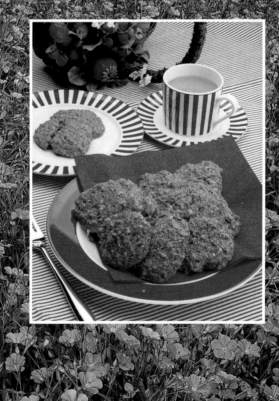

Siegfried's Favorite Breakfast

If I have to prepare a nourishing breakfast in a hurry, this is the one I like best. Not only does the kefir taste refreshingly good, but the ground flax seeds keep me from feeling hungry at least until noon.

1 cup (250 ml) **kefir or buttermilk**

2 tbsp freshly ground flax seeds

Put the flax seeds in an electric coffee grinder and pulse for 2 seconds. In a medium-size bowl, combine the flax seeds and the kefir and enjoy. Makes a perfect breakfast when served after a fresh fruit salad.

Serves 1

Variation

Add a sliced banana or in-season berries, a grated apple, kiwis, mango or any other fresh fruit.

Quark Muesli

Once you start eating freshly made muesli for breakfast you will never look back. This one is easy to prepare, provides high-value protein, essential fatty acids, complex carbohydrates, and enzymes for easy digestion. Kids will love this healthy breakfast!

½ cup of hazelnuts, walnuts or almonds

5 tbsp flax oil

1 grated apple, preferably Granny Smith or Macintosh

1 tbsp honey

1 cup quark

Grind the nuts in a blender. In a medium-size bowl combine nuts, oil, apple, honey and quark. Blend at low speed.

Serves 2

What is Quark?

Quark is the milk solid that separates from the whey when soured milk, kefir or yogurt is heated to 165°F (75°C) and poured through a strainer or cheesecloth. Quark has the consistency of soft cream cheese and can be used in sweet recipes with honey and fruit or in salty dishes with chives, herbs and seasoning salt. Alternatively it can be used as a spread, dip and dressing or as a filling for perogies or cheesecake. Whichever way you choose, quark is delicious. Quark can sometimes be substituted with cottage cheese. The difference is that quark is made from fermented (soured) milk in a low heat process while cottage cheese is made from sweet milk and rennet at a higher temperature.

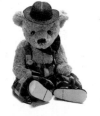

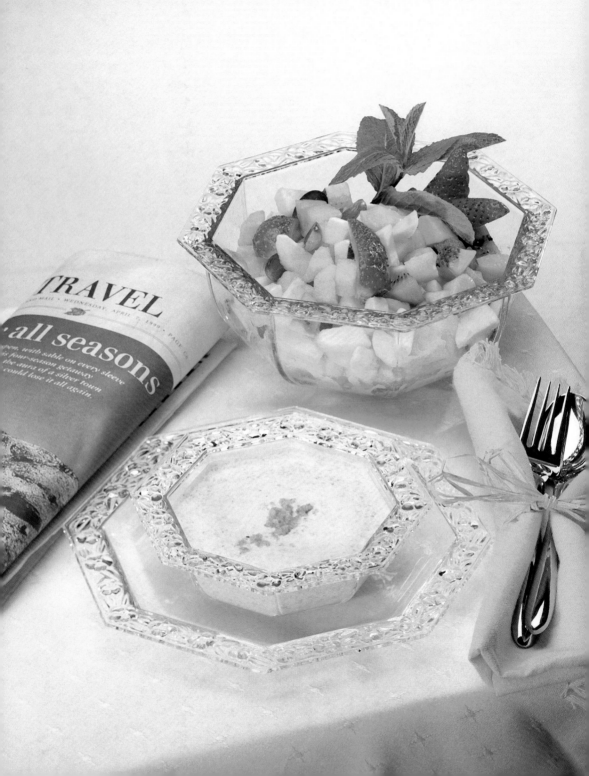

Budwig Muesli – the Original

This is a classic. Dr. Budwig introduced this particular recipe in her famous "Oil-Protein Diet" to combat cancer. It is popular all over Europe because it tastes so good, consists of mostly raw ingredients and is easily prepared.

1 cup quark or kefir cheese (or creamy cottage cheese which is made by whipping it in a blender)

½ cup (125 ml) buttermilk or kefir

1 tbsp honey

2 tbsp flax oil

2 tbsp ground flax seeds

1 grated apple

1 tbsp finely grated hazelnuts or walnuts

In a large bowl, blend the quark, buttermilk, honey and flax oil with a fork until creamy.

Spread a layer of ground flax in two breakfast bowls and cover with the grated apple and ground nuts. Finally, top with the smooth quark-oil blend and serve.

Serves 2

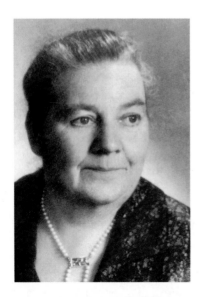

Dr. Johanna Budwig was a pioneer in the field of health and nutrition. She is perhaps best known for her research into the vital role of essential fatty acids, especially flax oil, in the treatment of cancer and other degenerative diseases. She was nominated for a Nobel prize as a result of this research.

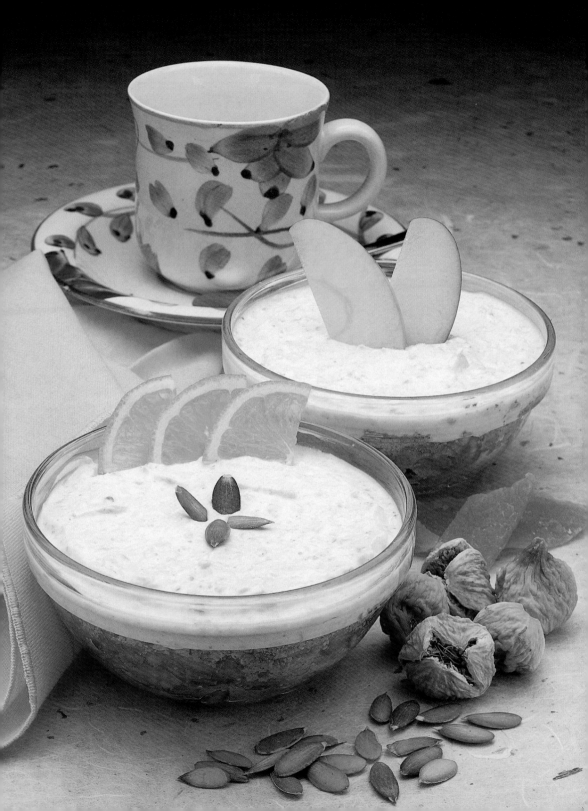

Rumpelstiltskin

Even though this recipe appears in the breakfast section, you can serve it as a dessert or a late night snack. It is easily digested, contributes to a good night's sleep and keeps your intestines healthy. Rumpelstiltskin can be prepared well ahead of time so you can make it in the evening and have it for breakfast. It is a pleasant taste surprise for anyone who eats it for the first time.

6 tbsp flax seeds, preferably the yellow variety

2 cups (500 ml) **milk**

2 tbsp ground hazelnuts

I banana, mashed with a fork

I tbsp honey

Juice from I orange

I apple, peeled, cored and diced

Pulse the flax seeds in an electric coffee grinder for 2 seconds. Bring the milk to a boil then stir in the flax meal. Boil for 30 seconds, remove from heat then pour into a bowl and let cool. This mixture will have the consistency of pudding. Add the ground nuts, the banana, honey and the orange juice. Whisk vigorously or blend on lowest speed in a blender. Fold in the apple and serve in glass bowls or parfait glasses.

Serves 4

Variation 1
When served as dessert, top with whipping cream and strawberries or kiwis. Everyone will enjoy this heavenly concoction.

Variation 2
You can add finely chopped dried and soaked fruits, dates, figs, raisins, prunes or pineapples to the pudding.

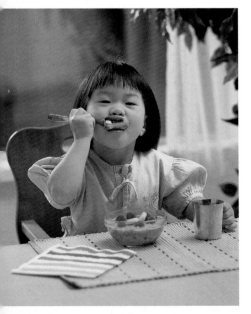

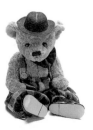

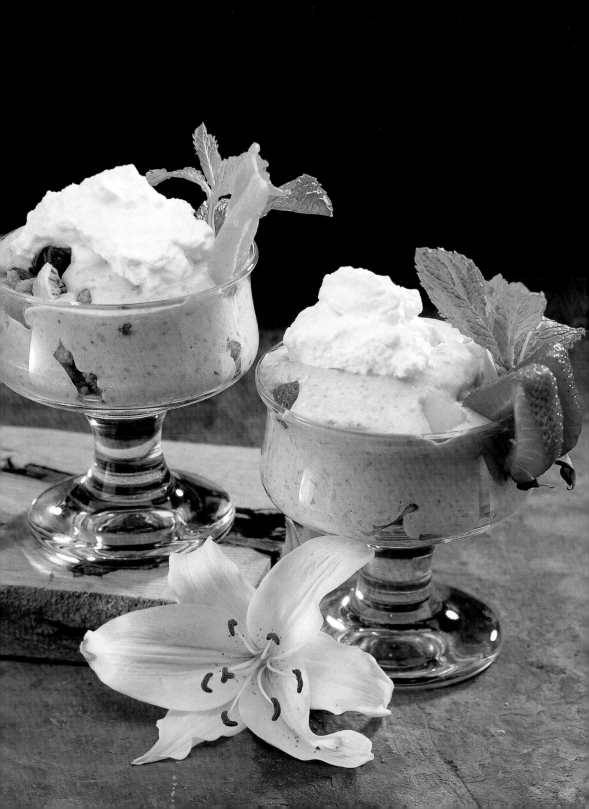

Kefir Quark with Flax Oil Dip

For a party lunch you may want to surprise your guests with this delicious new dip.

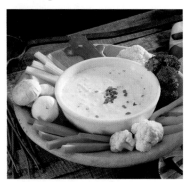

Quark with flax oil dip with vegetables

Keep the whey from this recipe – it makes a refreshing drink or it can be used in baking or in salad dressings.

Pour any amount of kefir into a glass jar and place the jar in a pot of boiling water until the milk solids separate from the whey. Pour the kefir solids through a fine mesh strainer or cheesecloth and let stand overnight. The next morning you will have the fresh-tasting creamy cheese known as quark.

Then, add a few tablespoons of kefir (or natural plain yogurt or buttermilk) to Quark with Flax Oil (see below). Add crushed garlic to taste. Serve as a dip for tomatoes, radishes, celery, carrots, broccoli or any other vegetables.

Variation

Add blue cheese to taste.

*Quark wi
flax
on brec*

Quark with Flax Oil

This traditional East German specialty is a tastier and healthier version of sour cream. It is delicious when served with baked potatoes, steamed carrots or corn. You can even carry it to work in a container and spread it on fresh rye bread, Swedish crisp bread or a cold baked potato.

I cup quark

4 tbsp flax oil

Herb seasoning salt to taste

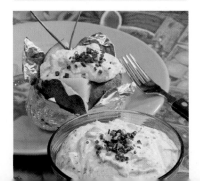

Combine all ingredients in a bowl and mix thoroughly.

Variation 1

Season the quark with fresh, finely chopped dill – the more dill, the better the flavor. Or add a generous amount of finely chopped chives to the quark for a surprisingly gratifying meal!

Variation 2

Grate fresh horseradish and mix it into the quark. The taste will be a surprise for your palate and the horseradish will act as an antibiotic for the urinary tract and kidneys and will even ease bladder discomfort.

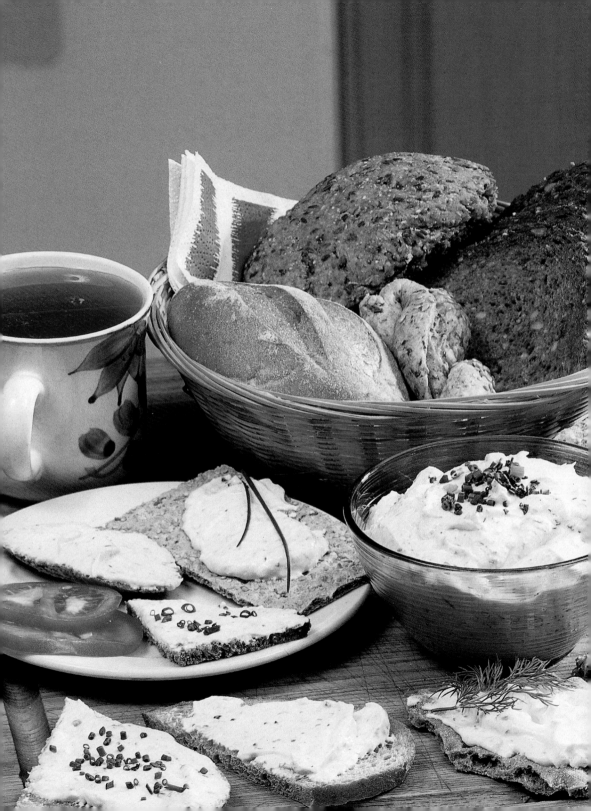

Coconut Butter Bread Spread

Many people want a tasty alternative to butter. I have experimented with a blend of coconut butter and flax oil and found it makes an extraordinary sandwich spread – especially with the addition of sautéed onions. The spread if kept refrigerated will stay fresh and will not go rancid for several months.

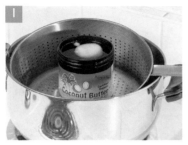

Place the coconut butter in a small container then set the container in a large bowl of warm water. This will soften the coconut butter and make it easier to work with. Be careful not to let the water run over the sides of the container.

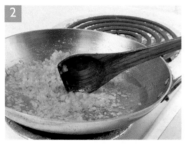

Pour ⅓ of the melted coconut butter into a saucepan over medium heat. Add chopped onion and salt and sauté, stirring constantly with a wooden spatula until the onions start to brown. Turn the heat down to low and carefully sauté the onions for a few more seconds without letting them burn.

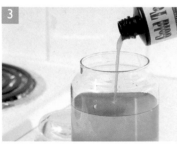

Remove from the heat, let cool to room temperature and then mix with the remaining coconut butter and the cold refrigerated flax oil. Pour into a container, seal tightly and place in the refrigerator. Turn the container upside down every ten minutes or stir the spread to prevent the onions from sinking to the bottom.

1¼ cups coconut butter

2 large onions, finely chopped

1 tsp sea salt

1 cup (250 ml) **flax oil**

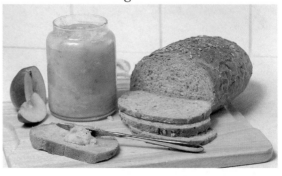

Try this spread on fresh rye bread with herbal salt. You'll love it.

Flax Oil-Enhanced Butter

If you live on your own it may not be practical to purchase a bottle of flax oil every three to four weeks as the oil can become rancid in this time. One way around this is to mix flax oil with butter to increase the butter's fatty acid profile. Any oil that is left over can be stored in the freezer as can the oil-enhanced butter.

I lb (450 g) **unsalted butter, at room temperature**

½ cup (125 ml) **flax oil**

In a medium-size bowl, blend the butter with the flax oil. The butter is now rich in omega-3 and omega-6 fatty acids and remains spreadable even when refrigerated. Do not use this enhanced butter for frying as heat destroys the essential fats. Use the flax oil-enhanced butter as a spread or a topping for baked potatoes or vegetables after they have been removed from the oven or stove.

Freshly Pressed Flax Oil Dip

Fresh sourdough rye bread, French bread or any other bread dipped in freshly pressed flax oil can be a simple yet very satisfying meal. For peasants in eastern Europe, this dish was part of their daily fare and was served with white or black radishes, which kept their livers and gall bladders in top shape.

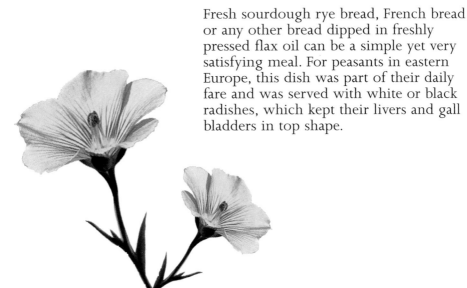

Basic Flax Oil Salad Dressing

A salad dressing is only as good as the ingredients used. If you want to have a superior dressing, use only the best ingredients – especially the oils. If you use any natural fermented vinegar such as balsamic, wine or apple cider vinegar, use them sparingly. If the flavor of any one ingredient dominates, you have used too much of it.

1 lemon, juice only

4 tbsp flax oil

1 tsp Maggi, soy sauce or Bragg's Aminos

2 tbsp minced onion

½ tsp mixed dry salad herbs

Chopped green onions (optional)

Beat lemon juice and flax oil until creamy. Stir in the Maggi and onions then add the herbs.

Use the basic flax oil dressing for butter lettuce or tender leaf lettuce.

Finely grated carrots topped with the basic flax oil dressing makes an appetizing salad.

Serves 4

Roquefort or Blue Cheese Dressing

The perfect dressing for a robust salad of leafy greens will beat anything you may have been served at a restaurant. Starting out with the *Basic Flax Oil Salad Dressing* makes all the difference. This is a treat for gourmet palates.

Basic Flax Oil Salad Dressing

3 tbsp genuine Roquefort or blue cheese, crumbled

6 tbsp kefir or 3 tbsp sour cream

2 tbsp nutritional yeast flakes (available from health food stores)

1 tsp red or white wine vinegar or apple cider vinegar

1 large clove garlic, minced

½ tsp dried Italian herbs

Combine all ingredients in a bowl and mix thoroughly.

This cheese dressing lends itself to salads made with mixed leafy greens, with cucumbers, tomatoes, carrots, green and red peppers.

Serves 6–8

Cucumber Salad with Dill Dressing

If there is any vegetable that can be improved with a dill dressing, it's the long English cucumber. Flax oil, kefir and dill is an excellent flavor combination.

2 cups English cucumbers

½ cup kefir or plain natural yogurt

2 tbsp flax oil

¼ tsp sea salt or herb salt

I bunch finely chopped fresh dill or I tbsp dried dillweed

Grate, chop, slice or dice cucumbers — whichever way you prefer, with or without peel, and mix with the other ingredients.

Serves 4

Kefir Dressing

You will have to look long and hard for a commercial dressing that is suitable for all salads. The following, however, is a "Jack-of-all-salads" that contains lactic acid (from the kefir) which makes the salad easy to digest.

Basic Flax Oil Salad Dressing (replace the dried Italian herbs with I bunch finely chopped fresh dill or I tsp dried dillweed)

6 tbsp kefir

I tbsp nutritional yeast flakes

Combine all ingredients in a bowl mix thoroughly.

Serves 4

You can only create an excellent salad if you use high-quality ingredients. The most important ingredient is a natural, unrefined fresh oil, like flax, walnut, hazelnut, pistachio or pumpkin seed oil. These are all very flavorful and rich in omega-3 and omega-6 essential fats. For a variety of flavors, combine flax and any of the other oils. Never heat these oils. For typical Greek or Italian dishes you can even mix flax with extra-virgin olive oil. It mellows the strong taste of the olive oil flavor.

Classic Mayonnaise with Flax Oil

Mayonnaise as an excellent healthy food has fallen from grace because of the inferior ingredients used in commercial preparations, such as white vinegar, and refined oils and sugar. This recipe puts mayonnaise back on its pedestal.

I egg yolk (from a free-range egg)

¾ cup (180 ml) **flax oil**

I tsp Dijon mustard

I tsp white wine vinegar or apple cider vinegar

I tsp freshly squeezed lemon juice

White pepper, garlic salt and herbal salt to taste

Place the egg yolk in a blender. Add oil very slowly and blend on the lowest speed until the mixture has a creamy consistency. Add mustard, vinegar and lemon juice then season to taste.

Baked Potatoes with Flax Oil

This simple recipe comes from eastern Europe. It is most popular in Siberia and East Germany where most families enjoy it several times each month. It is very easy to prepare.

4 medium baked potatoes

Bottle of fresh flax oil on the table

Herb salt

Crumble the baked potato with a fork then drizzle generously with flax oil and herb salt. Serve with vegetables of your choice. (Fresh, uncooked sauerkraut is the best!)

Serves 4

Avocado Dressing

With a little imagination you can create wonderful varieties of the *Basic Flax Oil Dressing*.

Basic Flax Oil Salad Dressing

I avocado

Add one soft, mashed avocado to the *Basic Flax Oil Salad Dressing*. This dressing is suitable for more robust salad greens like endive, romaine or a crunchy organic spring mix.

Serves 4

Raw Sauerkraut Salad with Flax Oil

Raw sauerkraut is one of the best vegetable sources of lactic acid, which is very beneficial for intestinal health. It can be bought in health food stores and delicatessens but the best sauerkraut is the kind you make at home. See *The Cultured Cabbage* by Klaus Kaufmann for simple instructions for homemade sauerkraut. Only unrefined flax seed oil will make this dish a delicacy.

2 cups raw sauerkraut
  (such as Eden brand)

2 tbsp onion, finely chopped

2 medium-size dill pickles, finely chopped

4 tbsp flax oil

Chopped parsley for garnish

Chop the sauerkraut into short strands then add onion and dill pickle and mix with flax oil. Garnish with parsley and serve.

Serves 4

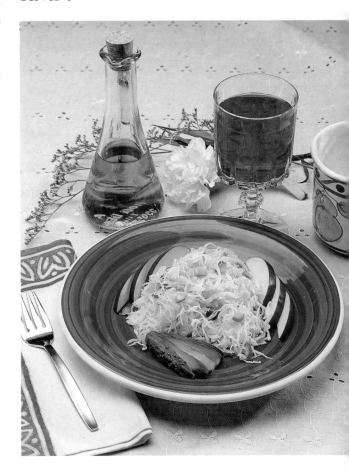

Flax and Miso Soup

When guests arrive unexpectedly, you can create this tasty soup in minutes.

1 tbsp butter

1 medium onion, diced

4 cups (1 liter) **water**

2 tbsp miso

1 vegetable bouillon cube (available at health food stores)

6 tbsp flax seeds, freshly ground (flax meal)

1 bunch fresh chives or parsley, finely chopped

Heat the butter in a large soup pot then sauté the onions until transparent. Add water. Dissolve miso and vegetable bouillon cube in the water then bring to the boil. Add the flax meal. After one minute remove from heat, garnish with chives and serve.

Serves 4

Flax and Vegetable Soup

This quick and nourishing vegetable soup can be prepared in fifteen minutes or less.

1 tbsp butter

1 medium onion, diced

4 cups (1 liter) **water**

1 tbsp miso

2 vegetable bouillon cubes (available at health food stores)

2 cups frozen vegetables, mixed carrots, peas, corn

4 to 6 tbsp (depending on desired consistency) **flax seeds, freshly ground** (flax meal)

Heat the butter in a soup pot then sauté the onion until transparent. Add the water then bring to the boil. Add all remaining ingredients except the herbs to the boiling water in the sequence listed to the left. After adding the flax meal, boil only for one minute, remove from heat and add chives or parsley before serving.

Serves 3–4

3 tbsp fresh herbs, chives or parsley, finely chopped

Miso Soup (front)
and Vegetable Soup (back)

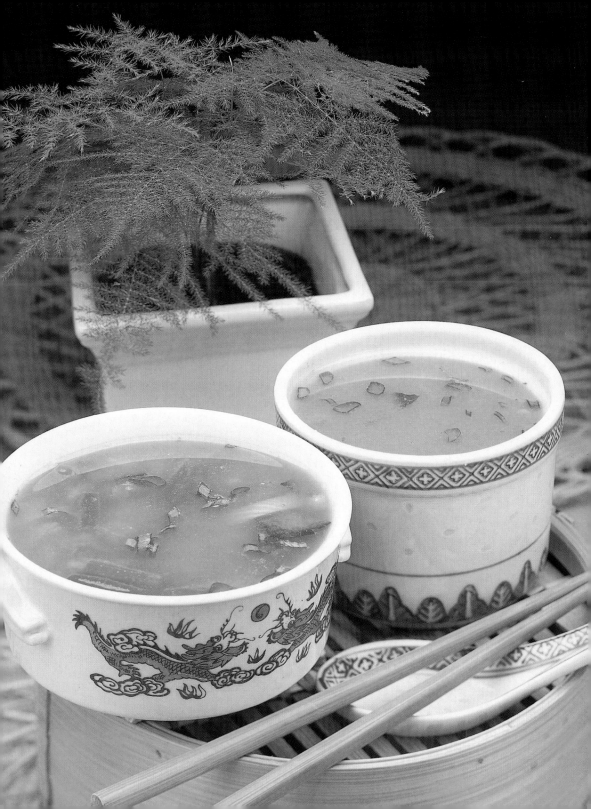

Potato Salad with Flax Oil

There are probably as many different recipes for potato salad as there are chefs in the world. This one I learned from my mother and my wife Christel loves it. It's her standby when catering company functions.

8 medium-size Yukon Gold potatoes (or nugget)

5 free-range eggs

Juice of 1 lemon

1 tsp apple cider vinegar or balsamic vinegar

4 tbsp flax seed oil

1 tbsp pumpkin seed oil

1 tbsp walnut oil (optional)

1 tsp vegetable broth powder

½ tsp vegetable salt

½ tbsp soy sauce or Maggi

1 medium size onion, finely chopped

1 clove garlic, minced

4 dill pickles, cut in ¼" cubes

Top of 1 tomato

Parsley for garnish

1 radish

Cook the potatoes in a large pot of boiling water until they are done but still firm, about thirty-five minutes; let cool. Cook the eggs in a medium-size pot of boiling water for three to four minutes. The yolks should still be soft.

In a large bowl, make a mayonnaise: combine the lemon juice, vinegar, oils, vegetable broth powder, salt and soy sauce. Whisk until creamy. Add the onion and garlic and mix thoroughly. Season to taste with more vegetable salt.

Peel the potatoes and cut them into thin slices. Add them to the mayonnaise along with the pickles.

Decorate with tomato, parsley and radish. Let sit for several hours in a cool place but don't refrigerate. This allows time for all the flavors to blend together.

Serves 6

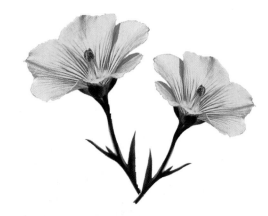

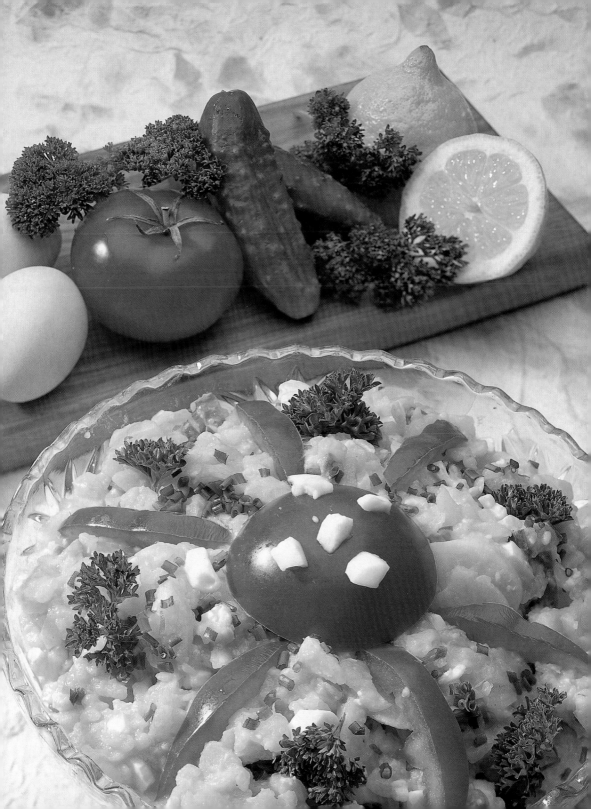

Flax Seed Bread

Commercially baked flax seed bread doesn't even compare with this traditional recipe.

1 cup whole flax seeds

1 cup ground flax seeds (flax meal)

¾ cup (180 ml) **hot water**

2 cups rye flour, coarsely ground

2 cups whole-wheat flour

1 oz (30 g or 1 heaping tbsp) **fresh yeast or 1 packet self rising dry yeast**

1 tbsp dried cane sugar, e.g. Sucanat or Rapadura

1 tbsp sea salt

3 tbsp unrefined almond, sesame, or extra-virgin olive oil

1 cup (250 ml) **lukewarm kefir or buttermilk**

Coconut butter for oiling the baking sheet

Preheat oven to 400°F (200°C).

Soak flax seeds in hot water for one hour. Once they have cooled, add flax meal and set aside. Using the kneading hook of your food processor, mix coarse rye flour and wheat flour then all other ingredients saving the ground flax for last. Start on lowest speed and increase to high speed and knead for approximately 5 minutes until the dough is smooth and all ingredients are entirely combined.

Cover the bowl and set in a warm place. When the volume has increased by at least half, set the dough on a lightly floured surface and knead thoroughly, adding small amounts of flour until firm. Form into an oval loaf, place on an oiled baking sheet, and let rise once more in a warm spot for about ½ hour or until it has noticeably increased in size. With a sharp knife, make several incisions on top of the loaf (don't squeeze) and brush with water.

Bake for one hour. For a crunchy crust, brush the bread several times with water while it is in the oven.

In conventional baked goods, flax meal can be substituted for shortening or cooking oil at a ratio of 3 to 1. For example, 1½ cups of ground flax can replace ½ cup of shortening, margarine or cooking oil. In order to derive the health benefits of flax it is important that no trans-fatty acids are present in these recipes. Therefore, under no circumstances should you use vegetable shortening, margarine or refined cooking oils. The oils which are heat-stable and suitable for baking are (in order of suitability) natural unrefined coconut butter, almond oil, olive oil and sesame oil.

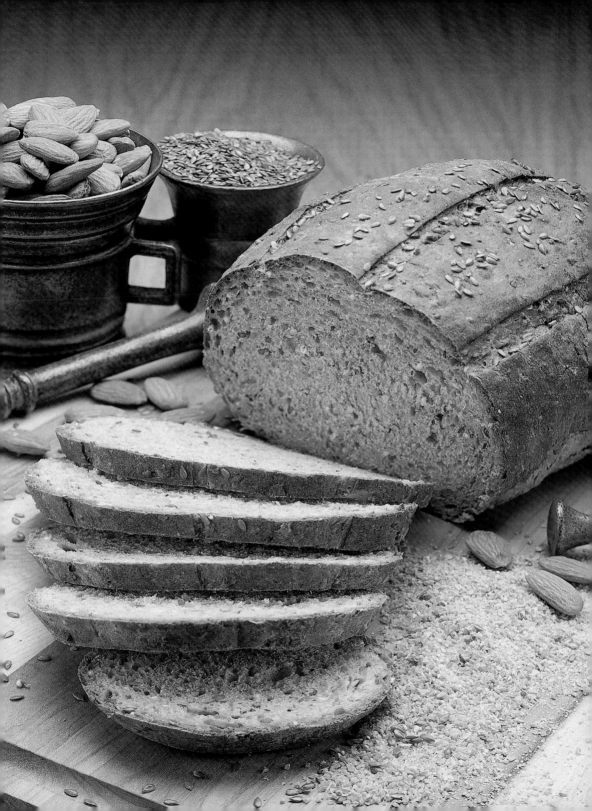

Flax Seed Buns

Bake lots of these and have them on hand when unexpected company comes around. They'll love them!

3 tbsp whole flax seeds

I cup (250 ml) plus 2 to 3 tbsp lukewarm milk

I oz (30 g) fresh yeast

2 tbsp kefir

I tsp sugar

3 tbsp freshly ground flax seeds (flax meal)

2 cups whole-wheat flour

2 tbsp almond oil, butter or coconut butter

I ½ tbsp sea salt

I cup unbleached white flour

I tbsp golden flax seeds for decoration

Coconut butter for oiling the baking sheet

Preheat oven to 400°F (200 °C).

Soak the whole flax seeds for one hour in half the milk then set aside. Stir the yeast, kefir and sugar into the remaining milk and keep in a warm place.

Measure flax meal and whole-wheat flour into a large bowl, make a well in the center and pour the yeast mixture into the well. Cover and let stand for ten minutes. Add the soaked flax seeds, almond oil or butter and salt, and mix thoroughly with a wooden spoon or the kneading hook of your food processor until smooth. Then turn out onto a floured surface and knead, adding small amounts of unbleached white flour at a time until the dough is firm but not sticky. Form a roll and cut into 16 equal sections. Form each part into a ball and place onto an oiled double-based baking sheet. Cover with a floured cloth and let rise for 20 minutes in a warm place. Using a sharp knife, cut a slit in the top of each bun, brush with milk and sprinkle with flax seeds.

Bake for 25 minutes. Remove from the oven and let cool on a cake rack. For freezing, let cool for at least 6 hours then place in a plastic bag and freeze. Frozen buns will keep for 1 month. Let thaw for 1 hour at room temperature.

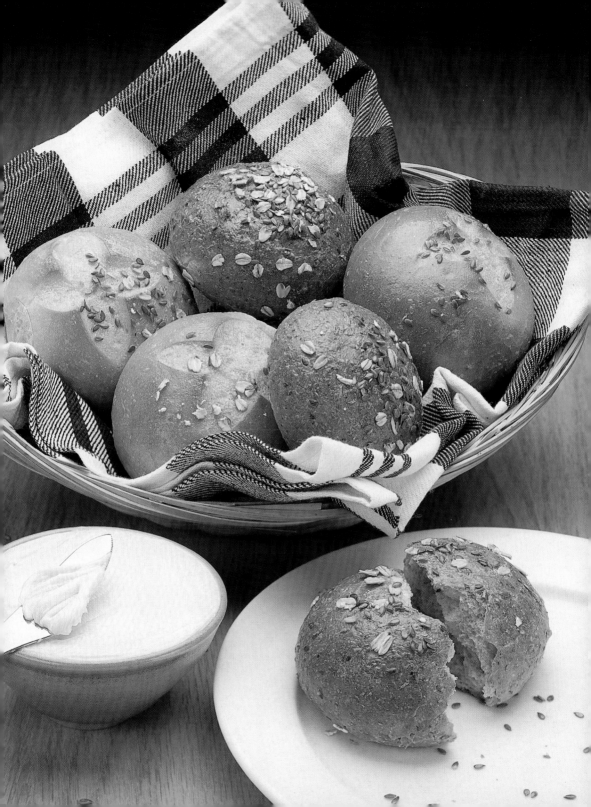

Flax-Almond Whole-Wheat Cookies

Kids love the tastes and textures of the flax seeds and almonds in this healthy cookie.

½ cup whole flax seeds

I cup (250 ml) kefir or buttermilk

I cup butter at room temperature

2 cups dried cane sugar e.g. Sucanat or Rapadura

2 eggs

2 tbsp pure vanilla extract

2 cups whole-wheat flour

½ cup ground flax seeds (flax meal)

I cup oatmeal

I tsp baking soda

I tsp baking powder

½ tsp sea salt

2 cups freshly chopped almonds

In a medium-size bowl, soak whole flax seeds in kefir or buttermilk for 2 hours.

Preheat oven to 350°F (180°C).

In a separate bowl, cream the butter and dried cane sugar until fluffy. Add one egg at a time and beat the mixture until creamy then add the vanilla extract.

In another large bowl combine flour, flax meal, oatmeal, baking powder, baking soda and sea salt. Stir in the kefir-soaked flax seeds and the butter-egg mixture. Add almonds and mix well.

Form the dough into balls and place on a cookie sheet allowing 2 inches between each ball. Bake one sheet at a time for 15 minutes or until the cookies are golden. Remove them from the oven and shift the cookies to a cooling rack.

Yields 6 dozen cookies

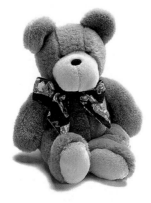

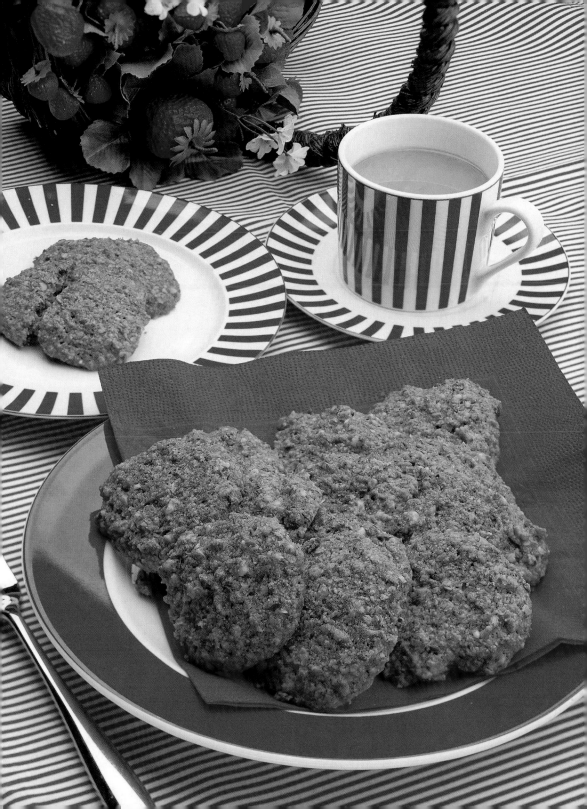

Flax Muffins with Chocolate Chips

Muffins are an American mainstay, but here is a recipe with an Old World twist.

½ cup whole flax seeds

1½ cups (375 ml) **kefir or buttermilk**

2 cups all-purpose flour

½ cup flax meal

½ cup dried cane sugar e.g. Sucanat or Rapadura

I tsp baking powder

2 tsp baking soda

½ tsp sea salt

2 eggs

¼ cup (60 ml) **almond oil or melted butter**

I tsp pure vanilla extract

I cup chocolate chips

Soak whole flax seeds in kefir for 2 hours. Preheat oven to 380°F (190°C).

In a large bowl, mix flour, flax meal, dried cane sugar, baking powder, baking soda and salt. In another bowl, beat eggs and combine with almond oil, vanilla and kefir-soaked flax seeds. Add the liquid ingredients to the dry ingredients and gently stir until smooth. Finally, fold in chocolate chips.

Pour the batter into 16 medium muffin cups so that they are no more than ¾ full, and bake for 20 minutes.

Let sit on a cooling rack for at least 5 minutes before serving.

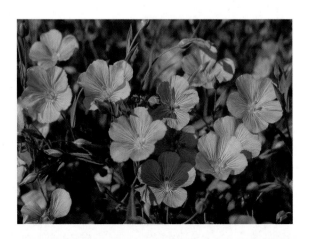

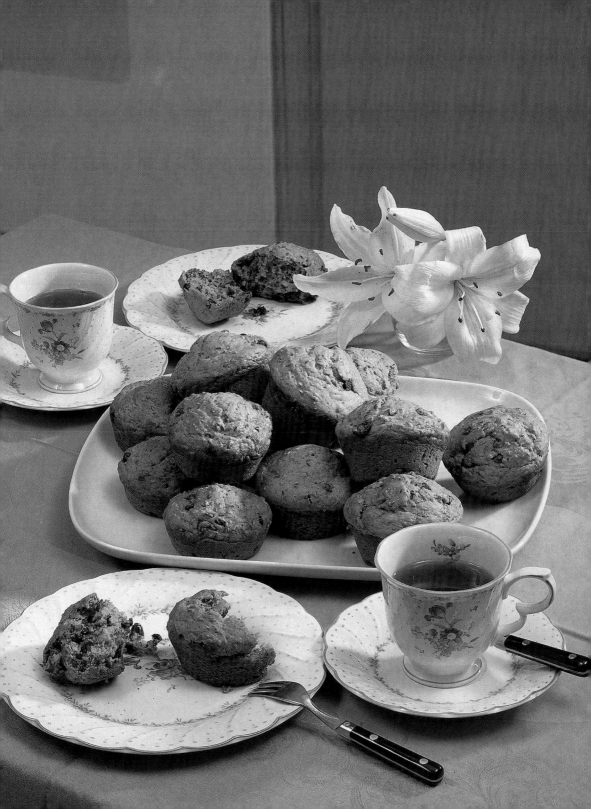

Fruit Flan in the Raw

This recipe is a contribution from friends who rave about it.

1 cup ground almonds

½ cup ground flax seeds (preferably golden flax seeds)

½ cup ground pine nuts

1 tbsp liquid Sucanat (pure cane syrup) **or pure maple syrup**

2 tbsp Rapadura sugar (dried sugar cane juice)

1 tbsp orange juice

1 tbsp lemon juice

Zest of ½ lemon

2 tbsp ground almonds

2 cups in-season fruit (preferably strawberries, raspberries or blueberries)

1 cup (250 ml) **whipping cream** (or the Creamy Coconut Topping to the right)

1 tbsp pure maple syrup

Combine the first 8 ingredients in a large bowl then form into a ball. Cover and refrigerate for ½ hour.

Sprinkle the bottom of a 9" pie shell with 2 tbsp ground almonds. Spread the dough into the pie shell to form an even crust and flute the edge of the crust with your fingers. Cover with plastic wrap and refrigerate for several hours.

Wash the fruit and slice it, if desired, then arrange the fruit decoratively on the pie crust.

Serve with *Creamy Coconut Topping*.

Creamy Coconut Topping:

Blend ingredients until creamy. Refrigerate for at least ½ hour for better consistency.

1 cup silken or soft tofu

2 tbsp coconut milk

2 tbsp maple syrup

1 tbsp lemon juice

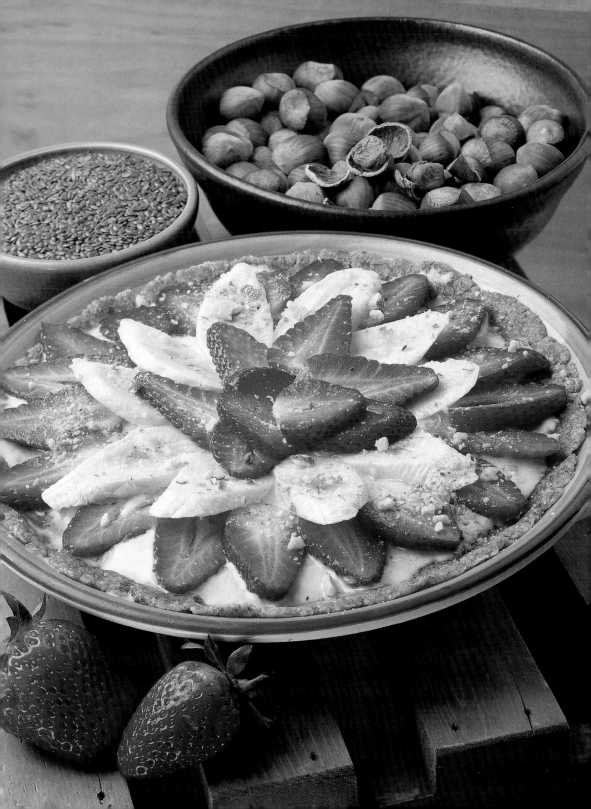

Hearty Whole-Wheat Flax Seed Bread for the Bread Machine

3 cups whole-wheat flour

5 tbsp whole flax seeds

2 tbsp freshly ground flax seeds

2 tbsp liquid honey

3 tsp gluten flour

2 tsp active dry yeast

1 tsp sea salt

2 tbsp unrefined sunflower or almond oil

1⅛ cup (270 ml) warm water in which to soak the flax seeds

All bread machines make bread in similar ways so you can safely follow the instructions on your bread machine.

When you program the machine you usually have to specify the weight of the loaf of bread you want to make. This recipe will make a 1-pound loaf. You will also have to specify the type of bread you want to make as bread machines have different settings. Here you should set the machine for a whole-wheat loaf.

Soak the whole flax seeds in the water for half an hour then proceed with the instructions on your bread machine.

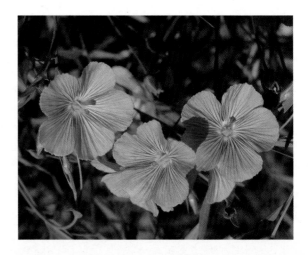

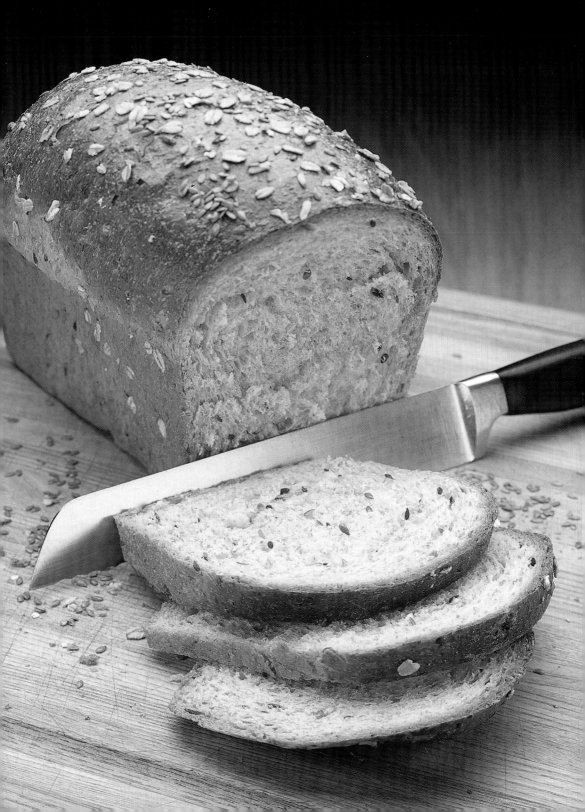

index

sources

Products available at health food stores

Flax Oil

Arrowhead Mills
110 South Lawton
Hereford, TX 79045

Barlean's
4936 Lake Terrell Road
Ferndale WA 982480
360–384–0485
800–445–3529

Flora
7400 Fraser Park Drive
Burnaby BC V5J 5B9
604–436–6000
800–663–0617 (Western Canada)
800–387–7541 (Eastern Canada)

Gold Top Organics
114423–37B Avenue
Edmonton AB T6J 0K2
780–483–1504

Jarrow Formulas
1824 South Robertson
Los Angeles CA 90035
310–204–6936
800–726–0886

Nature's Life
7180 Lampson Ave
Garden Grove CA 92841-3914
714–379–6500
800–854–6837 or 800–338–7979
www.nutritionexpress.com

Omega Nutrition of Canada, Inc.
1924 Franklin Street
Vancouver BC V5L 1R2
604–253–4677
800–661–3529
www.omegaflo.com

Flax Meal · · · · · · · · · · · · · · · · ·

Gold Top Organics
114423–37B Avenue
Edmonton AB T6J 0K2
780–483–1504

Omega Nutrition of Canada, Inc.
1924 Franklin Street
Vancouver BC V5L 1R2
800–661–3529
www.omegaflo.com

Omega–Life, Inc.
15355 Woodridge Road
Brookfield, WI 53005
414–786–2070
800–328–3529 (800–EAT–FLAX)

First published in 1999 by
alive books
7436 Fraser Park Drive
Burnaby BC V5J 5B9
604–435–1919
800–661–0303

Book Design: Paul Chau
Artwork: Terence Yeung
          Raymond Cheung
Photographs:
     Edmond Fong
     Siegfried Gursche
Editing:
     Paul Razzell
Copyediting:
     Julie Cheng
Food styling:
     Fred Edrissi
Recipes:
     Christel Gursche

Canadian Cataloguing in
Publication Data

Gursche, Siegfried, 1933 -
     Fantastic flax

(Alive natural health guides, 1
ISSN 1490-6503)
Includes index.
ISBN 1–55312–000–0

1. Flax–Health aspects 2. Cookery (Flax) I. Title. II. Series.
QK495.L74G87 1999
641.3'352   C99—910850—6

Printed in Canada

Revolutionary Health Books

alive Natural Health Guides

Each 64-page book focuses on a single subject, is written in easy-to-understand language and is lavishly illustrated with full color photographs.

New titles will be published every month in each of the four series.

Self Help Guides

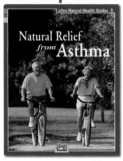

other titles to follow:

- **Nature's Own Candida Cure**
- **Natural Treatment for Chronic Fatigue Syndrome**
- **Fibromyalgia Be Gone!**
- **Heart Disease: Save Your Heart Naturally**
- **Liver Cleansing Diet**

Kitchen Guides

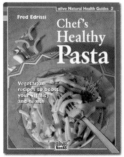

other titles to follow:

- **Baking with the Bread Machine**
- **Baking Bread: Delicious, Quick and Easy**
- **Healthy Breakfasts**
- **Salads and Salad Dressings**
- **Smoothies and Other Healthy Drinks**

Healing Foods & Herbs

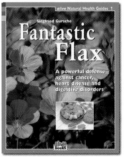

other titles to follow:

- **Calendula: The Healthy Skin Helper**
- **Ginkgo Biloba: The Good Memory Herb**
- **Rhubarb and the Heart**
- **Saw Palmetto: The Key to Prostate Health**
- **St. John's Wort: Sunshine for Your Soul**

Lifestyle & Alternative Treatments

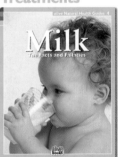

other titles to follow:

- **Maintain Health with Acupuncture**
- **The Complete Natural Cosmetics Book**
- **Kneipp Hydrotherapy at Home**
- **Magnetic Therapy and Natural Healing**
- **Sauna: Your Way to Better Health**

Vancouver
Canada

Great gifts at a great affordable price **$9.95 Cdn / $8.95 US / $11.95 Aust**

Natural Health Guides are available in bookstores and in health and nutrition centers. For information or to place orders please dial 800-663-6580 or 800-661-0303